Air Fryer Amazing Recipes

50+ Easy To Follow Air Fryer Recipes - From Breakfast To Dinner

Joana Smith

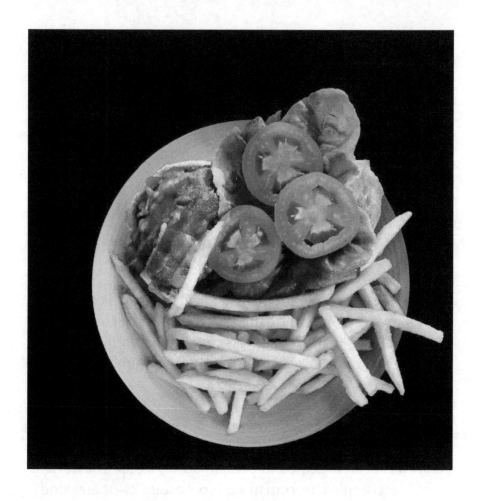

Table Of Contents

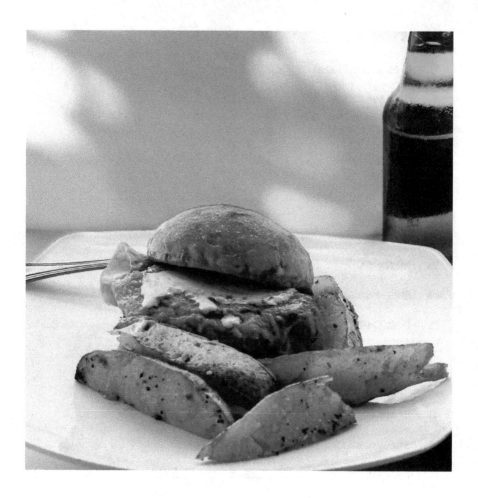

DESCRIPTION

The history of Air fryers dates back to a few years ago; exactly during the third quarter of the year 2010 and it was a completely revolutionary invention that was invented by Philips Electronics Company. Philips introduced the Air Fryer to the world and changed the conception of the culinary world all at once.

The Air Fryer is used as a substitute for your oven, stovetop, and deep fryer. It comes with various handy parts and other tools that you can buy to use your Air Fryer for different cooking styles, which include the following:

• Grilling. It provides the same heat to grill food ingredients without the need to flip them continuously. The hot air goes around the fryer, giving heating on all sides. The recipes include directions of how many times you ought to shake the pan during the cooking process.
To make the process of grilling faster, you can use a grill pan or a grill layer. They will soak the excess fat from the meat that you are cooking to give you delicious and healthy meals.

• Baking. The Air Fryer usually comes with a baking pan (or you can buy or use your own to make treats that are typically done using an oven. You can bake goodies, such as cakes, bread, cupcakes, muffins, and brownies in your Air Fryer.

• Roasting. It roasts food ingredients, which include vegetables and meat, faster than when you do it in the oven.

• Frying is its primary purpose – to cook fried foods with little or no oil.
You can cook most food items in an Air Fryer. There are some foods that you should refrain from cooking in the fryer because they will taste better when cooked in the traditional ways — they include fried foods with batter and steamed veggies, such as beans and carrots.

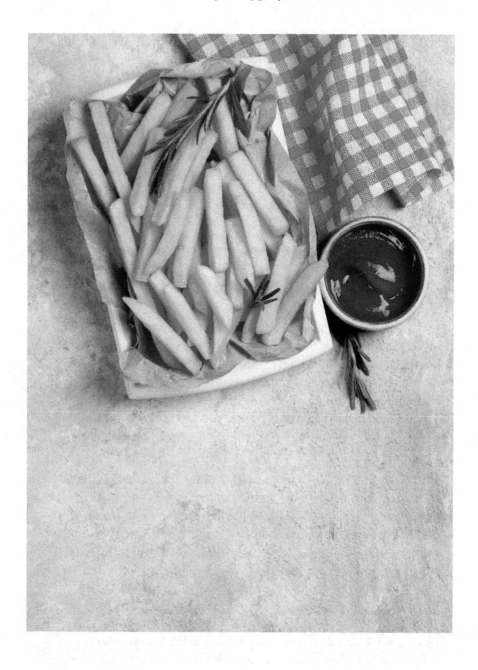

INTRODUCTION

There are many kinds of foods that you can cook using an air fryer, but there are also certain types that are not suited for it. Avoid cooking ingredients, which can be steamed, like beans and carrots. You also cannot fry foods covered in heavy batter in this appliance.

Aside from the above mentioned, you can cook most kinds of ingredients using an air fryer. You can use it to cook foods covered in light flour or breadcrumbs. You can cook a variety of vegetables in the appliance, such as cauliflower, asparagus, zucchini, kale, peppers, and corn on the cob. You can also use it to cook frozen foods and home prepared meals by following a different set of instructions for these purposes.

An air fryer also comes with another useful feature - the separator. It allows you to cook multiple dishes at a time. Use the separator to divide ingredients in the pan or basket. You have to make sure that all ingredients have the same temperature setting so that everything will cook evenly at the same time.

The Benefits of Air fryer

It is important to note that air fried foods are still fried. Unless you've decided to eliminate the use of oils in cooking, you must still be cautious about the food you eat. Despite that, it clearly presents a better and healthier option than deep-frying. It helps you avoid unnecessary fats and oils, which makes it an ideal companion when you intend to lose weight. It offers a lot more benefits, which include the following:

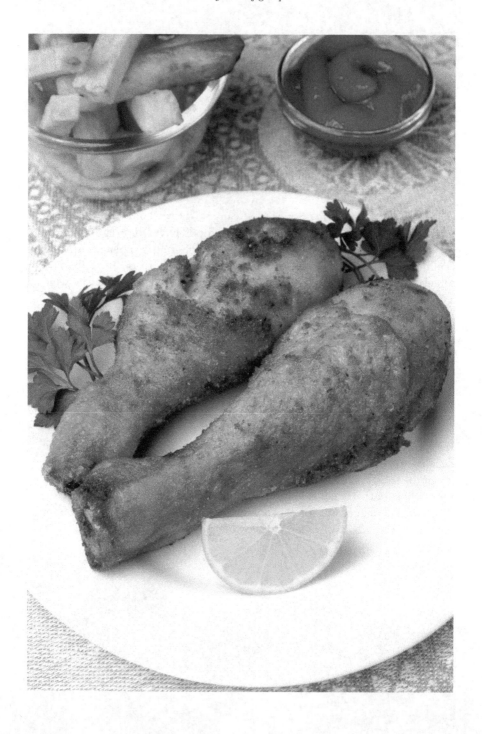

CHAPTER 1

BREAKFAST

1. Apple Cinnamon Pancakes

Preparation Time: 30 Minutes • Servings: 4

INGREDIENTS

- White flour-1¾ cups

- Sugar-2 tbsp.

- Baking powder-2 tsp.

- Vanilla extract -¼ tbsp.

- Cinnamon powder-2 tsp.

- Milk -1¼ cups

- Egg whisked -1

- Apple, peeled, cored and chopped-1 cup

- Cooking spray

DIRECTIONS

1. Mix everything in a bowl except cooking spray.

2. Grease the Air fryer's pan with cooking spray.

3. Pour ¼ of the batter in the Air fryer pan and place it in the Fryer.

4. Seal it and cook for 5 minutes at 360 o F.

5. Once cooked half way through then flip it.

6. Cook the remaining pancakes following the same steps.

7. Serve fresh.

NUTRITION: Calories: 172, Fat: 4g, Fiber: 4g, Carbs: 8g, Protein: 3g

2. Romanesco Tofu Quinoa

Preparation Time: 25 Minutes • Servings: 4

INGREDIENTS

- Firm tofu, cubed-12 ounces

- Maple syrup-3 tbsp.

- Soy sauce-¼ cup

- Olive oil -2 tbsp.

- Lime juice -2 tbsp.

- Fresh Romanesco, torn-1 pound

- Carrots, chopped-3

- Red bell pepper, chopped-1

- Baby spinach, torn-8 ounces

- Red quinoa, cooked-2 cups

DIRECTIONS

1. Toss tofu with maple syrup, oil, lime juice and soy sauce in a bowl.

2. Add this tofu to the Air fryer basket and seal it.

3. Cook for 15 minutes at 370 o F on Air fryer mode.

4. Shake it halfway through.

5. Once done, add the tofu to a bowl.

6. Add carrots, Romanesco, quinoa, bell pepper and spinach.

7. Mix well then serve.

8. Enjoy.

NUTRITION: Calories: 209, Fat: 7g, Fiber: 6g, Carbs: 8g, Protein: 4g

3. Mozzarella Avocado Mix

Preparation time: 5 minutes • Cooking time: 10 minutes

• Servings: INGREDIENTS

- 2 tablespoons butter, melted

- 1 cup avocado, peeled, pitted and cubed

- 1 cup black olives, pitted and sliced

- 1 cup mozzarella cheese, grated

- 1 tablespoon basil, chopped ½ teaspoon chili

  powder A pinch of salt and black pepper

DIRECTIONS

1. Preheat your Air Fryer at 360 degrees F, grease

   with the butter, add the avocado, olives and the

   other ingredients, toss, cook for 10 minutes,

   divide into bowls and serve for breakfast.

NUTRITION: Calories 207, Fat 14, Fiber 3, Carbs 4,

Protein 8

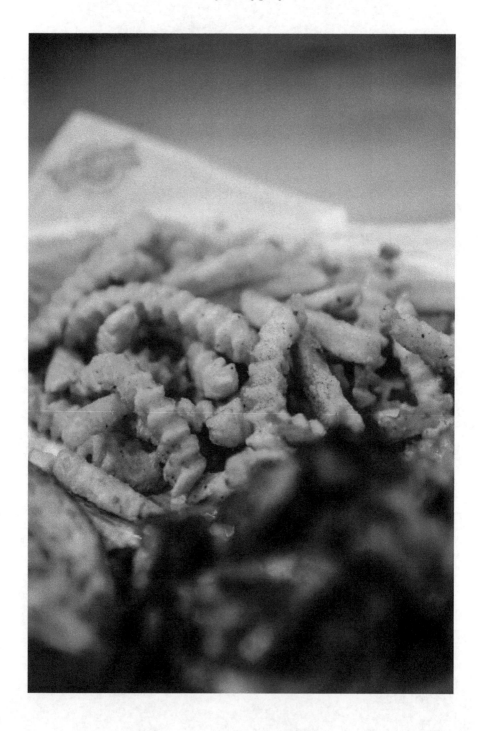

CHAPTER 2

MAINS

4. Shrimp Salad with Greens and Avocado

Preparation time: 10 minutes • Cooking time: 5 minutes •

Servings: 3

INGREDIENTS

- 8oz shrimps, peeled 1avocado, pitted

- 1cup fresh basil, chopped

- 1garlic clove, diced 1teaspoon olive oil

- 1teaspoon ground paprika

- 1teaspoon avocado oil

- 1cup fresh parsley, chopped

DIRECTIONS

1. Sprinkle the peeled shrimps with the olive oil

and ground paprika.

2. Stir the mixture.

3. Place the shrimps in the air fryer basket and cook them for 5 minutes at 400 F. Stir them after 3 minutes of cooking.

4. Meanwhile, peel the avocado and chop it.

5. Place the chopped avocado in the mixing bowl.

6. Add diced garlic and chopped fresh basil.

7. After this, add the chopped parsley and avocado oil.

8. Stir salad well.

9. When the shrimps are cooked – place them over the salad and serve immediately!

NUTRITION: Calories 252, Fat 16.2, Fiber 5.6, Carbs 9.1, Protein 19.5

5. Cauliflower Fritters with Carrot

Preparation time: 10 minutes • Cooking time: 10 minutes •

Servings: 6

INGREDIENTS

- 1-pound cauliflower head
- 1 carrot, grated
- 1 tablespoon almond flour
- 1 egg, beaten
- 1 tablespoon chopped dill
- 1 tablespoon chopped parsley
- ½ teaspoon salt
- 1 tablespoon olive oil
- ½ teaspoon chili flakes
- 1 tablespoon coconut flakes

DIRECTIONS

1. Chop the cauliflower and place it in the

blender.

2. Blend the cauliflower carefully.

3. Then place the blended cauliflower in the mixing bowl.

4. Add the grated carrot and almond flour.

5. After this, add the egg, chopped dill, chopped parsley, salt, coconut flakes, and chili flakes.

6. Stir the mixture carefully until smooth and homogenous.

7. Preheat the air fryer and pour the olive oil into the air fryer basket.

8. Then make the medium fritters from the cauliflower mixture with the help of the hands and place them in the air fryer basket.

9. Cook the fritters for 10 minutes at 400 F.

10. Turn the fritters into another side after 5

minutes of cooking.

11. When the fritters are cooked – chill them little.

12. Serve!

NUTRITION: Calories 85, Fat 5.8, Fiber 2.8, Carbs 6.5, Protein 3.7

6. Lamb Fillet with Tomato Gravy

Preparation time: 20 minutes • Cooking time: 10 minutes •

Servings: 3

INGREDIENTS

- 9oz lamb fillet

- 2tomatoes, chopped

- 1orange

- 1teaspoon salt

- 1tablespoon vinegar

- 1tablespoon avocado oil

- 1teaspoon chili flakes

- 11tablespoon almond flour

DIRECTIONS

1. Place the chopped tomatoes in the blender.

2. Peel the orange and add it to the blender too.

3. After this, add the salt, avocado oil, vinegar, chili

flakes, and almond flour.

4. Blend the mixture until smooth.

5. Then chop the lamb fillet roughly.

6. Pour the blended tomato mixture in the chopped lamb and stir it carefully.

7. Marinate the lamb fillet for 10 minutes.

8. After this, transfer the lamb fillet in the air fryer basket.

9. Sprinkle it with the remaining tomato mixture.

10. Cook the meat for 10 minutes at 400 F.

11. Stir the meat every 3 minutes.

12. When the meat is tender – transfer it in the serving bowls and sprinkle with the cooked gravy.

NUTRITION: Calories 262, Fat 11.7, Fiber 3.7, Carbs 12.7, Protein 27.3

7. Macaroni Cheese Toast

Cooking Time: 5 minutes • Servings: 2

INGREDIENTS

- 1egg, beaten 4tablespoons cheddar cheese, grated

- Salt and pepper to taste ½ cup macaroni and cheese

- 4bread slices

DIRECTIONS

1. Spread the cheese and macaroni and cheese over the two bread slices. Place the other bread slices on top of cheese and cut diagonally. In a bowl, beat egg and season with salt and pepper. Brush the egg mixture onto the bread. Place the bread into air fryer and cook at 300°Fahrenehit for 5-minutes.

NUTRITION: Calories: 250, Total Fat: 16g, Carbs: 9g, Protein: 14g

8. Cheese Burger Patties

Cooking Time: 15 minutes • Servings: 6

INGREDIENTS

- 1lb. ground beef

- 6cheddar cheese slices

- Pepper and salt to taste

DIRECTIONS

1. Preheat your air fryer to 390°Fahrenheit. Season beef with salt and pepper. Make six round shaped patties from the mixture and place them into air fryer basket. Air fry the patties for 10-minutes. Open the air fryer basket and place cheese slices on top of patties and place into air fryer with an additional cook time of 1-minute.

NUTRITION: Calories: 253, Total Fat: 14g, Carbs: 0.4g, Protein: 29g

9. Grilled Cheese Corn

Cooking Time: 15 minutes • Servings: 2

INGREDIENTS

- 2whole corn on the cob, peel husks and discard silk 1teaspoon olive oil

- 2teaspoons paprika

- ½ cup feta cheese, grated

DIRECTIONS

1. Rub the olive oil over corn then sprinkle with paprika and rub all over the corn. Preheat your air fryer to 300°Fahrenheit. Place the seasoned corn on the grill for 15-minutes. Place corn on a serving dish then sprinkle with grated cheese over corn. Serve and enjoy!

NUTRITION: Calories: 150, Total Fat: 10g, Carbs: 7g, Protein: 7g

CHAPTER 3

SIDES

10. Roast Butternut Pumpkin

Cooking Time: 20 minutes • Servings: 4

INGREDIENTS

- 1 butternut pumpkin, cut into 1-inch slices

- Sprigs of thyme for garnishing

- 2½ tablespoons toasted pine nuts

- Sea salt and pepper to taste

- 1½ tablespoons olive oil

- Vinaigrette:

- 6 tablespoons olive oil

- 1 tablespoon Dijon mustard

- Sea salt and black pepper to taste

- 2tablespoons balsamic vinegar

DIRECTIONS

1. Preheat air fryer to 390°Fahrenheit for 5-minutes. Cover the slices of pumpkin with olive oil and season with thyme, salt, and pepper. Set the air fryer to cook for 20-minutes, and place seasoned pumpkin slices into air fryer. Prepare the vinaigrette by combining all the vinaigrette ingredients in a bowl. Serve pumpkin covered with vinaigrette, sprinkle top with toasted pine nuts and sprigs of thyme.

NUTRITION: Calories: 257, Total Fat: 11.3g, Carbs: 10.6g, Protein: 8.3g

11. Parmesan Asparagus Fries

Cooking Time: 10 minutes • Servings: 5

INGREDIENTS

- 1lb. asparagus spears
- ¼ cup almond flour
- Salt and pepper to taste
- 2eggs, beaten
- ½ cup Parmesan cheese, grated
- 1cup pork rinds

DIRECTIONS

1. Preheat your air fryer to 380°Fahrenheit. Combine pork rinds and parmesan cheese in a small bowl. Season with salt and pepper. Line baking sheet with parchment paper. First, dip half the asparagus spears into flour, then into eggs, and finally into pork rind mixture. Place asparagus spears on the baking sheet

and bake for 10- minutes. Repeat with remaining spears.

NUTRITION: Calories: 20, Total Fat: 0.1g, Carbs: 3.9g, Protein: 2.2g

CHAPTER 4

SEAFOOD

12.Basil Swordfish Fillets

Preparation Time: 17 minutes • Servings: 4

INGREDIENTS

- 4swordfish fillets; boneless

- 2tbsp. butter; melted

- 1tbsp. olive oil

- 2tsp. basil; dried

- ¾ tsp. sweet paprika

- Juice of 1 lemon

DIRECTIONS

1. Take a bowl and mix the oil with the other

   ingredients except the fish fillets and whisk

2. Brush the fish with this mix, place it in your air fryer's basket and cook for 6 minutes on each side

3. Divide between plates and serve with a side salad.

NUTRITION: Calories: 216; Fat: 11g; Fiber: 3g; Carbs: 6g; Protein: 12g

13.Shrimp and Pesto

Preparation Time: 17 minutes • Servings: 4

INGREDIENTS

- 1½ lb. shrimp; peeled and deveined
- 1/3 cup pine nuts
- ½ cup olive oil
- ½ cup basil leaves
- ¼ cup parmesan; grated
- ½ cup parsley leaves
- 2tbsp. lemon juice
- ¼ tsp. lemon zest; grated
- A pinch of salt and black pepper

DIRECTIONS

1. In a blender, combine all the ingredients except the shrimp and pulse well. Take a bowl and mix the shrimp with the pesto and toss

2   Put the shrimp in your air fryer's basket and cook at 360°F for 12 minutes, flipping the shrimp halfway.

3.   Divide the shrimp into bowls and serve.

NUTRITION: Calories: 240; Fat: 10g; Fiber: 1g; Carbs: 4g; Protein: 12g

14.Honey Salmon

Preparation time: 5 minutes • Cooking time: 15 minutes

• Servings: 4 INGREDIENTS

- 4salmon fillets, boneless

- 2tablespoons lemon juice

- A pinch of salt and black pepper

- 1tablespoon honey

- 2tablespoons olive oil

- 2tablespoons chives, chopped

DIRECTIONS

1. In the air fryer's pan, mix the salmon with the lemon juice, honey and the other ingredients and cook at 350 degrees F for 15 minutes.

2. Divide the mix between plates and serve.

NUTRITION: Calories 272, Fat 8, Fiber 12, Carbs 15, Protein 16

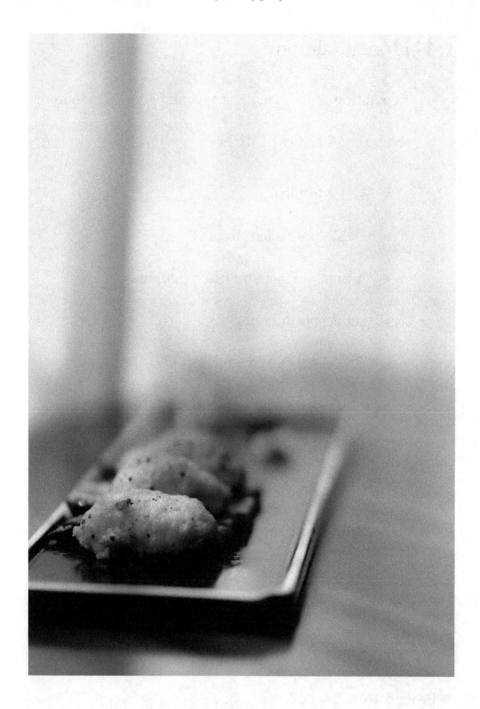

CHAPTER 5

POULTRY

15.Sriracha-vinegar Marinated Chicken

Servings: 4 • Cooking Time: 40 minutes

INGREDIENTS

- ¼ cup Thai fish sauce

- ¼ cups sriracha sauce

- ½ cup rice vinegar

- 1tablespoons sugar

- 2garlic cloves, minced

- 2pounds chicken breasts

- Juice from 1 lime, freshly squeezed

- Salt and pepper to taste

DIRECTIONS:

1. Place all Ingredients in a Ziploc bag except for the corn. Allow to marinate in the fridge for at least 2 hours.

2. Preheat the air fryer to 3900F.

3. Place the grill pan accessory in the air fryer.

4. Grill the chicken for 40 minutes and make sure to flip the chicken to grill evenly.

5. Meanwhile, place the marinade in a saucepan and heat over medium flame until it thickens.

6. Brush the chicken with the glaze and serve with cucumbers if desired.

NUTRITION: Calories: 427; Carbs: 6.7g; Protein: 49.1g; Fat: 22.6g

16.Chicken BBQ Recipe from Italy

Servings: 2 • Cooking Time: 40 minutes

INGREDIENTS

- 1tablespoon fresh Italian parsley

- 1tablespoon minced garlic

- 1-pound boneless chicken breasts

- 2tablespoons tomato paste

- Salt and pepper to taste

DIRECTIONS:

1. Place all Ingredients in a Ziploc bag except for the corn. Allow to marinate in the fridge for at least 2 hours. Preheat the air fryer to 3900F.

2. Place the grill pan accessory in the air fryer.

3. Grill the chicken for 40 minutes.

NUTRITION: Calories: 292; Carbs: 6.6g; Protein: 52.6g; Fat: 6.1g

17.Chili, Lime & Corn Chicken BBQ

Servings: 4 • Cooking Time: 40 minutes

INGREDIENTS

- ½ teaspoon cumin

- 1tablespoon lime juice

- 1teaspoon chili powder

- 2chicken breasts

- 2chicken thighs

- 2cups barbecue sauce

- 2teaspoon grated lime zest

- 4ears of corn, cleaned

- Salt and pepper to taste

DIRECTIONS:

1. Place all Ingredients in a Ziploc bag except for the corn. Allow to marinate in the fridge for at least 2 hours.

2. Preheat the air fryer to 3900F.

3. Place the grill pan accessory in the air fryer.

4. Grill the chicken and corn for 40 minutes.

5. Meanwhile, pour the marinade in a saucepan over medium heat until it thickens.

6. Before serving, brush the chicken and corn with the glaze.

NUTRITION: Calories per serving:849 ; Carbs: 87.7g; Protein: 52.3g; Fat: 32.1g

18.Chicken and Coriander Sauce

Preparation time: 10 minutes • Cooking time: 25 minutes • Servings: 4

INGREDIENTS

- 2pounds chicken breast, skinless, boneless and sliced 1cup cilantro, chopped
- Juice of 1 lime
- ½ cup heavy cream
- 1tablespoon olive oil
- ½ teaspoon cumin, ground
- 1teaspoon sweet paprika
- 5garlic cloves, chopped
- 1cup chicken stock
- A pinch of salt and black pepper

DIRECTIONS

1. In a blender, mix the cilantro with the lime juice

and the other ingredients except the chicken and the stock and pulse well.

2   Put the chicken, stock and sauce in the air fryer's pan, toss, introduce the pan in the fryer and cook at 380 degrees F for 25 minutes.

3. Divide the mix between plates and serve

NUTRITION: Calories 261, Fat 12, Fiber 7, Carbs 15, Protein 25

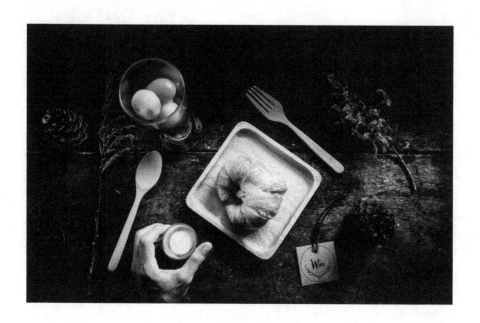

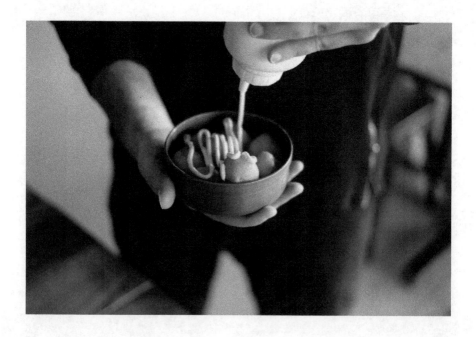

CHAPTER 6

MEAT

19. Greek Beef Mix

Preparation time: 5 minutes • Cooking time: 30 minutes

• Servings: 4

INGREDIENTS:

- 2pounds beef stew meat, roughly cubed

- 1teaspoon coriander, ground

- 1teaspoon garam masala

- 1teaspoon cumin, ground

- A pinch of salt and black pepper

- 1cup Greek yogurt

- ½ teaspoon turmeric powder

DIRECTIONS

1. In the air fryer's pan, mix the beef with the coriander and the other ingredients, toss and cook at 380 degrees F for 30 minutes.

2. Divide between plates and serve.

NUTRITION: Calories 283, Fat 13, Fiber 3, Carbs 6, Protein 15

20.   Beef and Fennel

Preparation time: 5 minutes • Cooking time: 30 minutes

• Servings: 4

INGREDIENTS

- 2pounds beef stew meat, cut into strips

- 2fennel bulbs, sliced

- 2tablespoons mustard

- A pinch of salt and black pepper

- 1tablespoon black peppercorns, ground

- 2tablespoons balsamic vinegar

- 2tablespoons olive oil

DIRECTIONS

1. In the air fryer's pan, mix the beef with the fennel and the other ingredients.

2. Put the pan in the fryer and cook at 380 degrees for 30 minutes.

3. Divide everything into bowls and serve.

NUTRITION: Calories 283, Fat 13, Fiber 2, Carbs 6,

Protein 17

21.Lamb and Eggplant Meatloaf

Preparation time: 5 minutes • Cooking time: 35 minutes

• Servings: 4

INGREDIENTS

- 2pounds lamb stew meat, ground

- 2eggplants, chopped

- 1yellow onion, chopped

- A pinch of salt and black pepper

- ½ teaspoon coriander, ground

- Cooking spray

- 2tablespoons cilantro, chopped

- 1egg

- 2tablespoons tomato paste

DIRECTIONS

1. In a bowl, mix the lamb with the eggplants of

   the ingredients except the cooking spray and

stir.

2. Grease a loaf pan that fits the air fryer with the cooking spray, add the mix and shape the meatloaf.

3. Put the pan in the air fryer and cook at 380 degrees F for 35 minutes.

4. Slice and serve with a side salad.

NUTRITION: Calories 263, Fat 12, Fiber 3, Carbs 6, Protein 15

CHAPTER 7

VEGETABLES

22.   Mini Cheesecake

Preparation Time: 25 minutes • Servings: 2

INGREDIENTS

- 4oz. full-fat cream cheese; softened.

- ⅛ cup powdered erythritol

- 1large egg.

- ½ cup walnuts

- 2tbsp. granular erythritol.

- 2tbsp. salted butter

- ½ tsp. vanilla extract.

DIRECTIONS

1. lace walnuts, butter and granular erythritol in a

food processor. Pulse until ingredients stick together and a dough form

2. Press dough into 4-inch springform pan then place the pan into the air fryer basket.

3. Adjust the temperature to 400 Degrees F and set the timer for 5 minutes. When timer beeps, remove the crust and let cool

4. Take a medium bowl, mix cream cheese with egg, vanilla extract and powdered erythritol until smooth.

5. Spoon mixture on top of baked walnut crust and place into the air fryer basket. Adjust the temperature to 300 Degrees F and set the timer for 10 minutes. Once done, chill for 2 hours before serving

NUTRITION: Calories: 531; Protein: 11.4g; Fiber: 2.3g; Fat: 48.3g; Carbs: 31.4g

23.   Cheesy Beets

Preparation time: 5 minutes • Cooking time: 30 minutes •

Servings: 4

INGREDIENTS

- 2beets, peeled and roughly cut into wedges

- 1cup mozzarella, shredded

- 1red onion, sliced

- A pinch of salt and black pepper

- 1tablespoon lemon juice

- 2tablespoons chives, chopped

- 2tablespoons olive oil

DIRECTIONS

1. In the air fryer's basket, mix the beets with the onion and the other ingredients except the cheese, toss and cook at 380 degrees F for 30 minutes.

2. Divide the corn between plates and serve with

cheese on top.

NUTRITION: Calories 140, Fat 4, Fiber 3, Carbs 5,

Protein 7

24. Frying Potatoes

Preparation time: 5 minutes • Cooking time: 40 minutes

• Servings: 4

INGREDIENTS

- 5to 6 medium potatoes

- Olive oil in a spray bottle if possible

- Mill salt

- Freshly ground pepper

DIRECTION:

1. Wash the potatoes well and dry them.

2. Brush with a little oil on both sides if not with

   the oil

3. Crush some ground salt and pepper on top.

4. Place the potatoes in the fryer basket

5. Set the cooking at 190°C for 40 minutes, in the

   middle of cooking turn the potatoes for even

cooking on both sides.

6. At the end of cooking, remove the potatoes from the basket, cut them in half and slightly scrape the melting potato inside and add only a little butter, and enjoy!

NUTRITION: Calories 365 Fat 17g Carbohydrates 48g Sugars 0.3g Protein 4g Cholesterol 0mg

CHAPTER 8

SNACKS

25.   Taco Cucumber Chips

Preparation time: 15 minutes • Cooking time: 3 Hours

• Servings: 4

INGREDIENTS

- 4cups very thin cucumber slices

- 2Tbsp apple cider vinegar

- 2tsp sea salt

- 2tsp taco seasoning

DIRECTIONS:

1. Preheat your air fryer to 200 degrees F.

2. Place the cucumber slices on a paper towel and layer
   another paper towel on top to absorb the moisture

in the cucumbers.

3. Place the dried slices in a large bowl and toss with the vinegar, taco seasoning, and salt.

4. Place the cucumber slices on a tray lined with parchment and then bake in the air fryer for 3 hours. The cucumbers will begin to curl and brown slightly.

5. Turn off the air fryer and let the cucumber slices cool inside the fryer (this will help them dry a little more).

6. Enjoy right away or store in an airtight container.

NUTRITION: Calories 23, Total Fat 0g, Saturated Fat 0g, Total Carbs 4g, Net Carbs 3g, Protein 1g, Sugar 2g, Fiber 1g, Sodium 38mg, Potassium 0g

26. Sweet Cauliflower Rice Dish

Preparation Time: 50 Minutes • Servings: 8

INGREDIENTS

- 3garlic cloves; minced
- 1cauliflower head; riced
- 1Whisked egg
- Drained water chestnuts-9-ounce
- Peas-3/4 cup
- Grated Ginger-1 tbsps
- Juice from ½ lemon
- Soy sauce-4 tbsps
- Peanut oil-1 tbsps
- Sesame oil-1 tbsps
- Chopped mushrooms-15-ounce

DIRECTIONS

1. Combine and mix cauliflower rice with peanut

oil, sesame oil, soy sauce, garlic, ginger and lemon juice in your air fryer; stir well.

2. Cover with lid and cook for 20 minutes at a temperature of 350°F.

3. Put chestnuts, peas, mushrooms, and egg; toss and cook for another 20 minutes at a temperature of 360°F.

4. Share among plates and serve for breakfast

27.   Tasty Hassel-Back Potatoes

Preparation Time: 30 Minutes • Servings: 2

INGREDIENTS

- Sweet paprika-½ tsp

- Olive oil - 2 tbsps

- 2potatoes peeled and thinly sliced almost all

  the way horizontally

- Dried oregano-½ tsp

- Dried basil-½ tsp

- Minced Garlic-1 tsp

- Seasoning- Salt and black pepper to the taste

DIRECTIONS

1. Combine and mix oil with garlic, salt, pepper,

   oregano, basil, and paprika in a bowl and whisk

   really well

2. Grease potatoes with this mix, place them in

your air fryer's basket and fry them for 20 minutes at a temperature of 360°F.

3. Share between plates and serve.

28.   Maple Broccoli Crunch

Preparation time: 5 minutes • Cooking time: 6 Hours •

Servings: 4

INGREDIENTS

- 4cups broccoli florets, chopped into bite sized pieces
- 1Tbsp olive oil
- 1tsp sea salt
- 1½ tsp maple extract

DIRECTIONS:

1. Preheat your air fryer to 135 degrees F.

2. Wash and drain the broccoli florets.

3. Place the broccoli in a large bowl and toss with the olive oil, maple extract, and sea salt.

4. Add the broccoli to the basket of your air fryer or spread them in a flat layer on the tray of your

air fryer (either option will work!).

5. Cook in the air fryer for about 6 hours, tossing the broccoli every hour or so to cook evenly. Essentially, you will be dehydrating the broccoli.

6. Once the broccoli is fully dried, remove it from the air fryer and then let cool. It will keep crisping as it cools.

7. Enjoy fresh or store in an airtight container for up to a month.

NUTRITION: Calories 54, Total Fat 3g, Saturated Fat 0g, Total Carbs 3g, Net Carbs 1g, Protein 2g, Sugar 1g, Fiber 2g, Sodium 610mg, Potassium 0g

29.   Veggie Crunch

Preparation time: 5 minutes • Cooking time: 6 Hours •

Servings: 4

INGREDIENTS

- 2cups broccoli florets, chopped into bite sized

  pieces

- 2cups cauliflower florets, chopped into bite sized

  pieces

- 1Tbsp olive oil

- 1tsp sea salt

DIRECTIONS:

1. Preheat your air fryer to 135 degrees F.

2. Wash and drain the florets.

3. Place the florets in a large bowl and toss with the

   olive oil and sea salt.

4. Add the florets to the basket of your air fryer or

spread them in a flat layer on the tray of your air fryer (either option will work!).

5. Cook in the air fryer for about 6 hours, tossing the florets every hour or so to cook evenly. Essentially, you will be dehydrating the veggies.

6. Once the florets is fully dried, remove it from the air fryer and then let cool. It will keep crisping as it cools.

7. Enjoy fresh or store in an airtight container for up to a month.

NUTRITION: Calories 53, Total Fat 3g, Saturated Fat 0g, Total Carbs 3g, Net Carbs 1g, Protein 2g, Sugar 0g, Fiber 2g, Sodium 610mg, Potassium 0g

30.   Shrimp Snack

Preparation Time: 15 minutes • Servings: 4

INGREDIENTS

- 1lb. shrimp; peeled and deveined

- ¼ cup olive oil 3garlic cloves; minced

- ¼ tsp. cayenne pepper

- Juice of ½ lemon

- A pinch of salt and black pepper

DIRECTIONS

1. In a pan that fits your air fryer, mix all the ingredients, toss,

2. Introduce in the fryer and cook at 370°F for 10 minutes

3. Servings as a snack

NUTRITION: Calories: 242; Fat: 14g; Fiber: 2g;

Carbs: 3g; Protein: 17g

31.Avocado Wraps

Preparation Time: 20 minutes • Servings: 4

INGREDIENTS

- 2avocados, peeled, pitted and cut into 12 wedges

- 1tbsp. ghee; melted

- 12bacon strips

DIRECTIONS

1. Wrap each avocado wedge in a bacon strip, brush them with the ghee.

2. Put them in your air fryer's basket and cook at 360°F for 15 minutes

3. Servings as an appetizer

NUTRITION: Calories: 161; Fat: 4g; Fiber: 2g; Carbs: 4g; Protein: 6g

32.   Cheesy Meatballs

Preparation Time: 30 minutes • Servings: 16 meatballs

INGREDIENTS

- 1lb. 80/20 ground beef.

- 3oz. low-moisture, whole-milk mozzarella, cubed

- 1large egg.

- ½ cup low-carb, no-sugar-added pasta sauce.

- ¼ cup grated Parmesan cheese.

- ¼ cup blanched finely ground almond flour.

- ¼ tsp. onion powder.

- tsp. dried parsley.

- ½ tsp. garlic powder.

DIRECTIONS

1. Take a large bowl, add ground beef, almond flour, parsley, garlic powder, onion powder and egg. Fold ingredients together until fully combined

2. Form the mixture into 2-inch balls and use your thumb or a spoon to create an indent in the center of each meatball. Place a cube of cheese in the center and form the ball around it.

3. Place the meatballs into the air fryer, working in batches if necessary. Adjust the temperature to 350 Degrees F and set the timer for 15 minutes

4. Meatballs will be slightly crispy on the outside and fully cooked when at least 180 Degrees F internally.

5. When they are finished cooking, toss the meatballs in the sauce and sprinkle with grated Parmesan for serving.

NUTRITION: Calories: 447; Protein: 29.6g; Fiber: 1.8g; Fat: 29.7g; Carbs: 5.4g

33.   Tuna Appetizer

Preparation Time: 15 minutes • Servings: 2

INGREDIENTS

- 1lb. tuna, skinless; boneless and cubed

- 3scallion stalks; minced

- 1chili pepper; minced

- 2tomatoes; cubed

- 1tbsp. coconut aminos

- 2tbsp. olive oil

- 1tbsp. coconut cream

- 1tsp. sesame seeds

DIRECTIONS

1. In a pan that fits your air fryer, mix all the ingredients except the sesame seeds, toss, introduce in the fryer and cook at 360°F for 10 minutes

2. Divide into bowls and serve as an appetizer with sesame seeds sprinkled on top.

NUTRITION: Calories: 231; Fat: 18g; Fiber: 3g; Carbs: 4g; Protein: 18g

34.   Cheese and Leeks Dip

Preparation Time: 17 minutes • Servings: 6

INGREDIENTS

- 2spring onions; minced 4leeks; sliced

- ¼ cup coconut cream 3tbsp. coconut milk

- 2tbsp. butter; melted

- Salt and white pepper to the taste

DIRECTIONS

1. In a pan that fits your air fryer, mix all the ingredients and whisk them well.

2. Introduce the pan in the fryer and cook at 390°F for 12 minutes. Divide into bowls and serve

NUTRITION: Calories: 204; Fat: 12g; Fiber: 2g; Carbs: 4g; Protein: 14g

35.   Cucumber Salsa

Preparation Time: 10 minutes • Servings: 4

INGREDIENTS

- 1½ lb. cucumbers; sliced

- 2red chili peppers; chopped.

- 2tomatoes cubed 2spring onions; chopped.

- 1tbsp. balsamic vinegar

- 2tbsp. ginger; grated

- A drizzle of olive oil

DIRECTIONS

- In a pan that fits your air fryer, mix all the ingredients, toss, introduce in the fryer and cook at 340°F for 5 minutes

- Divide into bowls and serve cold as an appetizer.

NUTRITION: Calories: 150; Fat: 2g; Fiber: 1g; Carbs: 2g; Protein: 4g

36.   Chicken Cubes

Preparation Time: 25 minutes • Servings: 4

INGREDIENTS

- 1lb. chicken breasts, skinless; boneless and cubed
- 2eggs
- ¾ cup coconut flakes
- 2tsp. garlic powder
- Cooking spray
- Salt and black pepper to taste.

DIRECTIONS

1. Put the coconut in a bowl and mix the eggs with garlic powder, salt and pepper in a second one.

2. Dredge the chicken cubes in eggs and then in coconut and arrange them all in your air fryer's basket

3. Grease with cooking spray, cook at 370°F for 20 minutes. Arrange the chicken bites on a platter and serve as an appetizer.

NUTRITION: Calories: 202; Fat: 12g; Fiber: 2g; Carbs: 4g; Protein: 7g

37.   Salmon Spread

Preparation Time: 11 minutes Servings: 4

INGREDIENTS

- 8oz. cream cheese, soft ½ cup coconut cream

- 4oz. smoked salmon, skinless; boneless and minced 2tbsp. lemon juice

- 1tbsp. chives; chopped.

- A pinch of salt and black pepper

DIRECTIONS

1. Take a bowl and mix all the ingredients and whisk them really well.

2. Transfer the mix to a ramekin, place it in your air fryer's basket and cook at 360°F for 6 minutes

NUTRITION: Calories: 180; Fat: 7g; Fiber: 1g; Carbs: 5g; Protein: 7g

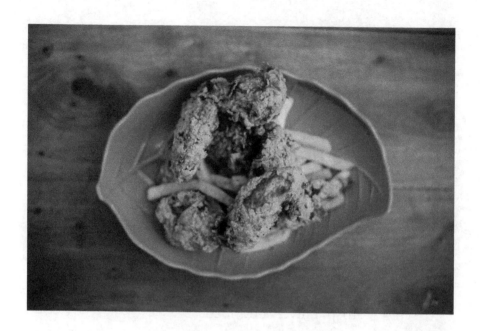

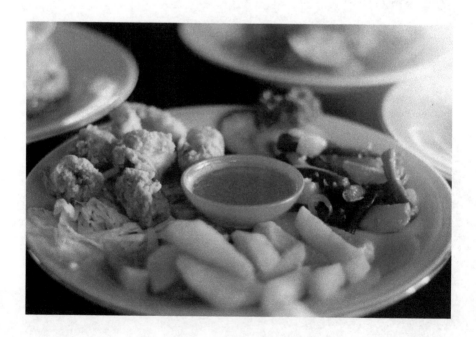

CHAPTER 9

DESSERT

38.   Olives Spread

Preparation time: 5 minutes • Cooking time: 5 minutes •

Servings: 6

INGREDIENTS

- 1cup black olives, pitted and chopped

- 1cup kalamata olives, pitted and chopped

- 1cup green olives, pitted and chopped

- 1cup Greek yogurt

- 1tablespoon olive oil

- 3tablespoons lemon juice

- 1cup basil, chopped

- A pinch of salt and black pepper

DIRECTIONS

1. In a blender, combine the olives with the yogurt and the other ingredients, pulse well and transfer to a ramekin.

2. Place the ramekin in your air fryer's basket and cook at 350 degrees F for 5 minutes.

3. Serve as a party spread.

NUTRITION: Calories 120, Fat 5, Fiber 2, Carbs 3, Protein 7

39.   Melon Salsa

Preparation time: 5 minutes • Cooking time: 5 minutes •

Servings: 4

INGREDIENTS:

- 1cup watermelon, peeled and cubed

- 1cup cherry tomatoes, halved

- 1cup corn

- 1cup baby spinach

- 2spring onions, chopped

- 2tablespoons lime juice

- 1tablespoon avocado oil

- 2teaspoons parsley, chopped

- Cooking spray

DIRECTIONS

1. In the air fryer's pan, mix the watermelon with

   the tomatoes and the other ingredients and

toss.

2   Introduce the pan in the machine and cook at

360 degrees F for 5 minutes.

3.   Divide into bowls and serve as an appetizer.

NUTRITION: Calories 148, Fat 1, Fiber 2, Carbs 3, Protein 5

40.   Shrimp Spread

Preparation time: 5 minutes • Cooking time: 6 minutes •

Servings: 4

INGREDIENTS

- 1cup cream cheese, soft

- Juice of 1 lime Zest of 1 lime, grated

- 1pound shrimp, peeled, deveined and minced

- A pinch of salt and black pepper

- 1tablespoon chives, chopped

DIRECTIONS

1. In a bowl, mix all the ingredients, whisk them really well, transfer the mix to a ramekin, place it in your air fryer's basket and cook at 370 degrees F for 6 minutes.

2. Serve as a party spread.

NUTRITION: Calories 180, Fat 7, Fiber 1, Carbs 5, Protein 7

41.Pork Dip

Preparation time: 10 minutes • Cooking time: 20 minutes •

Servings: 4

INGREDIENTS

- 1pound pork stew meat, ground

- 1tablespoon olive oil

- 1red onion, chopped

- ¼ teaspoon rosemary, dried

- ½ teaspoon coriander, ground

- 1cup heavy cream

- 1tablespoon cilantro, chopped

- 2garlic cloves, minced

- A pinch of salt and black pepper

DIRECTIONS

1. Preheat the air fryer with the oil at 370 degrees

   F, add the meat and cook for 5 minutes.

2 Add the rest of the ingredients, cook for 15 minutes more, divide into bowls and serve as a party dip.

NUTRITION: Calories 249, Fat 16, Fiber 2, Carbs 3, Protein 17

42.   Spinach Dip

Preparation time: 6 minutes • Cooking time: 20 minutes • Servings: 6

INGREDIENTS

- 1cup cream cheese, soft 1cup mozzarella, shredded 2cups baby spinach

- 1cup heavy cream A pinch of salt and black pepper 2tablespoons butter, melted

DIRECTIONS

1. In the air fryer's pan, mix the cream cheese with the mozzarella and the other ingredients, put the pan in the machine and cook at 360 degrees F for 20 minutes.

2. Serve as a party dip.

NUTRITION: Calories 210, Fat 8, Fiber 1, Carbs 3, Protein 8

43. Pork and Spinach Bowls

Preparation time: 10 minutes • Cooking time: 20 minutes •

Servings: 6

INGREDIENTS

- 1pound pork stew meat, cut into strips

- 1cup baby spinach

- 1cup cherry tomatoes, halved

- 1tablespoon balsamic vinegar

- 2tablespoons olive oil

- 1teaspoon sweet paprika

- A pinch of salt and black pepper

- 1tablespoon chives, chopped

DIRECTIONS

1. In the air fryer's pan, mix the meat with the spinach and the other ingredients, put the pan in the machine and cook at 360 degrees F for 20 minutes.

2   Divide into bowls and serve as a snack.

NUTRITION: Calories 251, Fat 14, Fiber 3, Carbs 5,

Protein 18

44. Tomato and Radish Bowls

Preparation time: 5 minutes • Cooking time: 20

minutes • Servings: 6

INGREDIENTS

- 1pound cherry tomatoes, halved

- 2cups radishes, halved

- 1cup baby kale

- 1cup carrots, peeled and grated

- 1tablespoon olive oil

- Juice of 1 lime

- 2ounces watercress

- A pinch of salt and black pepper

- 1tablespoon chives, chopped

DIRECTIONS

1. In the air fryer's pan, mix the tomatoes
   with the radishes and the other ingredients,
   put the pan in the machine and cook at 360

degrees F for 20 minutes.

2   Divide into bowls and serve.

NUTRITION: Calories 131, Fat 7, Fiber 2, Carbs 4,

Protein 7

45.   Strawberry pie

reparation Time: 30 Minutes • Servings: 12

INGREDIENTS

- Coconut: 1 cup shredded

- Butter: ¼ cup

- Sunflower seeds: 1 cup

- Filling Ingredients:

- Gelatin: 1 tbsp

- Cream cheese: 8 oz.

- Lemon juice: ½ tbsp

- Ste-via: ¼ tbsp

- Strawberries: 4 oz.

- Water: 4 tbsp

- Heavy cream: ½ cup

- Strawberries: 8 oz. chopped for serving

DIRECTIONS

1. Mix sunflower seeds, coconut, a pinch of salt and butter in a food processor then pulse it

2. Press it on the bottom of your cake pan then heat the pan over medium heat

3. Slowly add gelatin and stir. Cook for a few minutes then leave it aside to cool

4. Place it to your food processor, and 4 oz. strawberries, cream cheese, lemon juice and Ste via. Blend it

5. Add heavy cream and stir.

6. Spread it over the crust top it with 4 oz. strawberries and cook in the air fryer for 15 minutes at 330 ° F

7. Keep it in the fridge, then serve when needed.

NUTRITION: Calories: 234; Fat: 23; Protein: 7;

Carbohydrates: 6; Fiber: 2

46. Grape Pudding

Preparation time: 10 minutes • Cooking time: 40 minutes • Servings: 6

INGREDIENTS:

- 1cup grapes curd
- 3cups grapes
- 3and ½ ounces maple syrup
- 3tablespoons flax meal combined with 3 tablespoons water
- 2ounces coconut butter, melted
- 3and ½ ounces almond milk
- ½ cup almond flour
- ½ teaspoon baking powder

DIRECTIONS

1. In a bowl, mix the half of the fruit curd with the grapes stir and divide into 6 heatproof

ramekins.

2. In a bowl, mix flax meal with maple syrup, melted coconut butter, the rest of the curd, baking powder, milk and flour and stir well.

3. Divide this into the ramekins as well, introduce in the fryer and cook at 200 degrees F for 40 minutes.

4. Leave puddings to cool down and serve!

5. Enjoy!

NUTRITION: Calories 230, Fat 22, Fiber 3, Carbs 17, Protein 8

47.   Coconut and Pumpkin Seeds Bars

Preparation time: 10 minutes • Cooking time: 35

minutes • Servings: 4

INGREDIENTS:

- 1cup coconut, shredded

- ½ cup almonds

- ½ cup pecans, chopped

- 2tablespoons coconut sugar

- ½ cup pumpkin seeds

- ½ cup sunflower seeds

- 2tablespoons sunflower oil

- 1teaspoon nutmeg, ground

- 1teaspoon pumpkin pie spice

DIRECTIONS

1. In a bowl, mix almonds and pecans with

   pumpkin seeds, sunflower seeds, coconut,

nutmeg and pie spice and stir well.

2. Heat up a pan with the oil over medium heat, add sugar, stir well, pour this over nuts and coconut mix and stir well.

3. Spread this on a lined baking sheet that fits your air fryer, introduce in your air fryer and cook at 300 degrees F and bake for 25 minutes.

4. Leave the mix aside to cool down, cut and serve.

5. Enjoy!

NUTRITION: Calories 252, Fat 7, Fiber 8, Carbs 12, Protein 7

48. Chocolate Cookies

Preparation time: 10 minutes • Cooking time: 25 minutes • Servings: 12

INGREDIENTS

- 1teaspoon vanilla extract
- ½ cup coconut butter, melted
- 1tablespoon flax meal combined with 2 tablespoons water
- 4tablespoons coconut sugar
- 2cups flour
- ½ cup unsweetened vegan chocolate chips

DIRECTIONS

1. In a bowl, mix flax meal with vanilla extract and sugar and stir well.

2. Add melted butter, flour and half of the chocolate chips and stir everything.

3. Transfer this to a pan that fits your air fryer, spread the rest of the chocolate chips on top, introduce in the fryer at 330 degrees F and bake for 25 minutes.

4. Slice when it's cold and serve.

5. Enjoy!

NUTRITION: Calories 230, Fat 12, Fiber 2, Carbs 13, Protein 5

49. Cinnamon Bananas

Preparation time: 10 minutes • Cooking time: 15 minutes • Servings: 4

INGREDIENTS

- 3tablespoons coconut butter
- 2tablespoons flax meal combined with 2 tablespoons water
- 8bananas, peeled and halved
- ½ cup corn flour
- 3tablespoons cinnamon powder
- 1cup vegan breadcrumbs

DIRECTIONS

1. Heat up a pan with the butter over medium-high heat, add breadcrumbs, stir and cook for 4 minutes and then transfer to a bowl.

2. Roll each banana in flour, flax meal and

breadcrumbs mix.

3. Arrange bananas in your air fryer's basket, dust with cinnamon sugar and cook at 280 degrees F for 10 minutes.

4. Transfer to plates and serve.

5. Enjoy!

NUTRITION: Calories 214, Fat 1, Fiber 4, Carbs 12, Protein 4

50.   Coffee Pudding

Preparation time: 10 minutes • Cooking time: 10 minutes • Servings: 4

INGREDIENTS

- 4ounces coconut butter

- 4ounces   dark vegan chocolate, chopped

- Juice of ½ orange

- 1teaspoon baking powder

- 2ounces whole wheat flour

- ½ teaspoon instant coffee

- 2tablespoons   flax meal combined with 2 tablespoons water

- 2ounces coconut sugar

DIRECTIONS

1. Heat up a pan with the coconut butter over medium

heat, add chocolate and orange juice, stir well and take off heat.

2 In a bowl, mix sugar with instant coffee and flax meal, beat using your mixer, add chocolate mix, flour, salt and baking powder and stir well.

3. Pour this into a greased pan, introduce in your air fryer, cook at 360 degrees F for

10 minutes, divide between plates and serve.

4. Enjoy!

NUTRITION: Calories 189, Fat 6, Fiber 4, Carbs 14, Protein 3

51.Cinnamon Cream

Preparation time: 10 minutes • Cooking time: 20 minutes • Servings: 4

INGREDIENTS:

- 1cup cream cheese, soft 1cup coconut cream
- ½ cup heavy cream 3tablespoons sugar
- 1and ½ tablespoons cinnamon powder
- 2eggs, whisked

DIRECTIONS

1. In the air fryer's pan, combine the cream cheese with the cream and the other ingredients, whisk well, cook at 350 degrees F for 20 minutes, divide into bowls and serve warm.

NUTRITION: Calories 200, Fat 11, Fiber 2, Carbs 15, Protein 4

52.   Pumpkin Bowls

Preparation time: 10 minutes • Cooking time: 15 minutes • Servings: 4 INGREDIENTS

- 2cups pumpkin flesh, cubed

- 1cup heavy cream

- 1teaspoon cinnamon powder

- 3tablespoons sugar

- 1teaspoon nutmeg, ground

DIRECTIONS

1. In a pan that fits your air fryer, combine the pumpkin with the cream and the other ingredients, introduce in the fryer and cook at 360 degrees F for 15 minutes.

2. Divide into bowls and serve.

NUTRITION: Calories 212, Fat 5, Fiber 2, Carbs 15, Protein 7

DAY MEAL PLAN

DAY	BREAKFAST	MAINS	DESSERTS
1.	Stuffed Portobello Mushrooms with Ground Beef	Indian Chickpeas	Butter Cookies
2.	Basil-Spinach Quiche	White Beans with Rosemary	Cream Cheese and Zucchinis Bars
3.	Stuffed Chicken Roll with Mushrooms	Squash Bowls	Coconut Cookies
4.	Eggs on Avocado Burgers	Cauliflower tew with Tomatoes and Green Chilies	Lemon Cookies
5.	Applesauce Mash with Sweet Potato	Simple Quinoa Stew	Delicious cheesecake
6.	Bacon and Kale Breakfast Salad	Green Beans with Carrot	Macaroons
7.	Fish Fritatta	Chickpeas and Lentils Mix	Amaretto and bread dough
8.	Spinach Frittata	Garlic Pork Chops	Orange cake
9.	Kale Quiche with Eggs	Honey Ginger Salmon	Apple bread

		Steaks	
10.	Olives Rice Mix	Mustard Pork Balls	Strawberry pie
11.	Sweet Quinoa Mix	Beef Meatballs in Tomato Sauce	Bread pudding
12.	Creamy Almond Rice	Green Stuffed Peppers	Pomegranate and chocolate bars
13.	Chives Quinoa Bowls	Sweet & Sour Chicken Skewer	Crisp apples
14.	Potato Casserole	Lamb Meatballs	Cocoa cookies
15.	Turkey and Peppers Bowls	Spiced Green Beans with Veggies	Strawberry shortcakes
16.	Turkey Tortillas	Chipotle Green Beans	Lentils and dates brownies
17.	Avocado Eggs Mix	Tomato and Cranberry Beans Pasta	Chocolate cookies
18.	Maple Apple Quinoa	Mexican Casserole	Mini lava cakes
19.	Chopped Kale with Ground Beef	Spicy Herb Chicken Wings	Banana bread
20.	Bacon Wrapped Chicken Fillet	Roasted Cauliflower with Nuts & Raisins	Granola
21.	Egg Whites with Sliced Tomatoes	Red Potatoes with Green	Tomato cake

		Beans and Chutney	
22.	Beef Balls with Sesame and Dill	Simple Italian Veggie Salad	Chocolate cake
23.	Zucchini Rounds with Ground Chicken	Spiced Brown Rice with Mung Beans	Coffee cheesecakes
24.	Meatball Breakfast Salad	Eggplant and Tomato Sauce	Fried banana
25.	Tomatoes with Chicken	Lemony Endive Mix	Banana cake
26.	Cherry Tomatoes Fritatta	Lentils and Spinach Casserole	Espresso cream and pears
27.	Whisked Eggs with Ground Chicken	Scallions and Endives with Rice	Lime cheesecakes Wrapped Pears
28.	Breakfast Bacon Hash	Cabbage and Tomatoes	Strawberry cobbler
29.	Eggplant and weet Potato Hash	Lemon Halibut	Almond and cocoa bars
30.	Eggs in Avocado	Medium-Rare Beef Steak	Ginger cheesecake
31.	Spaghetti Squash Casserole Cups	Fried Cod & Spring Onion	Plum cake